ARE YOU AN ASSET?

11 Keys To Being A Woman Who Brings
More To The Table Than Her Appetite

APRIL MASON

For permission requests, please contact:

info@aprilmason.com

ISBN **978-0-9891254-4-4**

Printed in USA

Table of Contents

Introduction...1

Chapter 1: Femininity 14

Chapter 2: Organization 22

Chapter 3: Service 27

Chapter 4: Finances 31

Chapter 5: Class 36

Chapter 6: Independence...............................41

Chapter 7: Health.....................................45

Chapter 8: Faith......................................52

Chapter 9: Wisdom.....................................58

Chapter 10: Entrepreneurship 62

Chapter 11: Self Love 69

Conclusion..76

Other Helpful Resources 77

INTRODUCTION

I was sitting in the audience at an awards ceremony, where thirty women were receiving awards for their outstanding achievements. As I sat there, I noticed something that became quite disturbing to me. One by one each lady came up, accepted her award, and her acceptance speech went a little something like this:

"I'd like to thank God, my children, friends, and family. Without them, none of this would've been possible".

Hmm, was it me or was something missing? Out of the thirty women, I noticed that only five of them actually thanked a spouse or significant other. As I looked around the room filled with about 700 women, I asked myself, "I wonder how many here are married?

Better yet, I wonder how many of these powerful, successful business, and career women are even dating?"

Now let's fast forward two years. I was nominated and won the award for Entrepreneur Innovator at the same event. In that moment it hit me, I am now in the same position as the women who received the award before me. How ironic is that? I must admit, that was a hard pill to swallow. To be honest, I thought I had it all together. I thought I was an Asset because of my list of accomplishments and my ability to be a strong woman. Isn't that what determines if I'll make a good mate or not? I decided that it was time to make some changes. For crying out loud, it wasn't like I was getting any younger. I put everything down for over 18 months to do some serious soul-searching. During my time of isolation, I had to ask myself the real hard question. It was time to figure out what I was doing wrong. I knew the only way to do that was to get down to who I am at my core, and what I truly desired.

Our society has continuously bombarded us with images of powerful, strong women, but most of them are single. Think about it, from politics to entertainment to everything in between. So now you have troupes of beautiful, powerful, successful, independent women who have been able to purchase their own homes, luxury cars, have good credit, money in the bank, educated, and man less. Congrats to you girl for making it happen. Wait! I forgot to mention, the little dogs. Oh, don't act like you don't know what I am talking about. The little dog that some women use as their companion instead of connecting with a man. Yeah, that dog. Now, before you get offended, let me be clear. In no way, shape, form or fashion am I saying that you should dumb down, not educate yourself, or secure financial wealth and material possessions. I am all about empowering yourself and being self-sufficient. I just don't want you to forget to take your femininity and womanly wiles with you. Yeah, I call it being self-sufficient and not independent. We'll discuss that a little later.

Now let me tell you what happened during my 18 months of isolation. Throughout my career, I have accomplished so many amazing things, graced stages across the country, appeared on television shows, wrote books, made a good living for myself and my children, worked hard, and became the strong woman that I was trained to be. You see, I would've never guessed that my path would've taken me down this road. Once I started telling my story of how I started my first business homeless with three kids, living in a shelter with $50 from a welfare check, how I overcame molestation, domestic violence, rape and low self-esteem, I started receiving calls from across the country to inspire and empower other women. I never set out for the world's definition of success. I never asked to be booked for events. I never sent out press kits. I never made phone calls pitching myself or any of that. People sought after me, and I was blessed in the process. However, one day something happened. Something on the inside of me clicked. Let me explain.

I went through an awful breakup. That breakup opened a part of me that I never knew was there. It was the core of who I am. It was my womanhood, my femininity. Even though the relationship ended on a sad note, it was the very thing I needed to realize that this part of me even existed. Sometimes what we believe is the worst thing that could have ever happened to us, turns out to be the best thing that could have ever happened. This incident started my transformation. I started feeling things that I had never felt before. The more time I spent with myself, I began to feel a sudden calmness, peace, and wanting to be one with nature. Throughout this process, I also learned the type of woman that I am. I began to realize that all the things that I had done over the years were only to feed my family. At that moment I realized that my "Why" in life had changed.

My children were graduating high school heading off to college, and I no longer had anyone to take care of. As I uncovered more and more gems about who I am, I sat back and asked myself, "April what do you really want? What makes you happy? What do you enjoy?". Having that time to myself was a tad difficult. This was because I was so programmed to do, do, do and go, go, go. Long story short, I realized that I am, and I enjoy being a domesticated woman. I love to take care of the home and those in it. One thing I discovered about my past relationships is, I enjoyed working with my mate. I enjoyed putting my energy into building our empire. I also enjoyed putting my time into building his platform as well. I know you may be thinking, "What about you and your dreams?" Therefore it's imperative to understand how you're wired. Some women are called to be a wife, mother, and a support system and they enjoy every moment of it. There are several types of women. I will call my kind of woman the amplifier.

My joy and happiness had always come from building up my family and others. This doesn't take away from me. I've done more at the age of 42 than most will do in a lifetime. Trust me, I'm good. Also, at any given time if I chose to get back out there, I can. I've just learned how to have a work-life balance. I've found myself being drawn to gardening, wanting to do arts and crafts, and DIY projects around my home. Candles everywhere, changed my decor to light from dark and color coordinated my closet. Learning how to sew was also something I wanted to do, I'm working on that. The deeper I looked within, the more I felt myself let the burdens on my shoulders drop to the floor. No more worrying about my image and the opinions of others. No more doing what I was "supposed" to do. No more operating from what "they" say the American Dream should be. I felt liberated so much, I started to walk slower and let the anxiety go. Heck, what have I been in a hurry for all these years anyway? I learned to say no and make no apologies for it. I learned how to put myself first. It was like the hand of the creator was molding me into the woman that I was always created to be. I no longer felt the need to be strong and carry it all. Even though I am a single parent and responsible for my family, I started to reposition my thinking.

For years, I was choosing to take on the mom and dad role. If you think about it, have you ever heard a man say, "I'm dad and mom?" Or, does he do what a father does, and have female friends or family handle the mom stuff? A man never tries to be both, but for some reason we do. No one asked us to, we just assume the responsibility. As women, we can never instill in our children what a man can. We just aren't equipped with the same set of information or genetic makeup.

Two of the main things I discovered during this process was, how you perceive things will determine the attitude you will have about them. As well as, how to do what was in my power, and not stress about the rest. As women, we are such nurtures and givers, I had to learn how to intentionally put myself in a position to receive. I began to let the men in my life be men. This included the bagger at the grocery store. When he would ask, "Do you need help to your car, Ma'am?", I started to say," Yes." Now, you already know as women our typical first response is, "I got it!" Well, I didn't want to have it anymore. When a man would ask if he could pump my gas, I would say "Yes." I didn't care if it was a homeless man on the street trying to make a buck, I still allowed him to do it to help me. My goal was to say yes more which in turn, help me rewire the years of society pushing the "be strong, you go girl, you can do it by yourself girl, you don't need a man girl" mentality. Just because you can do it alone or have been put in a position to do it alone, it doesn't mean it was designed to be that way.

Now I know you might be saying, "What if I don't want a man?" That's fine too. My message isn't for you. However, I have to ask you this, if Mr. Right came along at this very moment would you turn him away? You know, considering you said you don't want a man and all. I'm just saying, if you answered that you would turn him away, then I accept it. However, if your answer is "Well if the right man came along, heck no I won't turn him away," that means your statement is a defense mechanism. I know, I've been there and done that too. It comes from past negative experiences and being afraid to believe that there is someone great out there designed for you. It's kind of like trying to keep hope alive, but not believing that you can have a fulfilling relationship. This is our way of protecting ourselves, so we don't get hurt again. Now you and I both know that does not work. You can't want a thing and be afraid of receiving it at the same time. Don't get me wrong; I am not saying that you should get yourself together only to attract a man.

What I'm saying is, get yourself together for you. At that point, you can present yourself as an asset to someone else. Besides, let's not act like having a good man around doesn't bring a smile to our face and joy to our hearts. Honey, there is nothing like having someone to have around to put his muscles to use when you need to open a jar of pickles, fix the tire, and just say "Baby don't worry about it, I got it," and he really has it. Girl, I get excited just thinking about it. Okay, let me calm down and get back to the task at hand.

I believe that to become a high valued asset woman that you, you must get back to womanhood and femininity. I had to realize that being a smart and successful woman isn't what makes me valuable or an asset. Those are just added bonuses. With this understanding, I felt like I'm probably not the only woman who is going through awakening. I asked myself, "Who is the example of what the perfect balance looks like?", "Is there such a woman that has it all?" After searching high and low for the prototype, I found her. She doesn't have a name, but she does have a description.

Growing up I was raised a devout Christian. As an adult, I no longer practice religion, but I am heavily into spirituality. I often heard about this Proverbs 31 Woman. The menfolk would say "Wow, I just wish I could find a Proverbs 31 woman." My first thought would always be, "maybe you haven't found her because you haven't become what you're asking for, boo!" Let me stop right there, that's another book. The Proverbs 31 woman was described as the ultimate woman in the Christian community. Although this story is told in the bible, Christian and Non-Christian can take away valuable principles.

Check out what the bible says about her.

Proverbs 31:10 – 31 *"A wife of noble character who can find? She's worth far more than rubies. Her husband has full confidence in her and lacks nothing of value. She brings him good not harm all the days of her life. She selects wool and flax and works with her eager hands. She is like the merchant ships bringing her food from afar. She gets up while it is still dark. She provides food for her family and portions for her servant girls. She considers a field and buys it. Out of her earnings, she plants a vineyard. She sets about her work vigorously. He* *arms are strong for her task. She sees that her trading is profitable and her lamp does not go out at night. In her hands, she holds to the staff and grasps the spindle with her fingers. She opens her arms to the poor and extends her hand to the needy. When it snows, she has no fear for her household for all are clothed with scarlet. She makes coverings for her bed and clothed in fine linen and purple. Her husband is respected at the city gates where he takes his seat among the elders of the land. She makes linen garments and sells them and supplies the merchants with sashes. She is clothed with strength and dignity. She can laugh at the days to come. She speaks with wisdom, and faithful instruction is on her tongue.*

She watches over her affairs of her household and does not eat of the bread of idleness. Her children arise and call her blessed. Her husband also, and he praises her. Many women do noble things, but you surpass them all. Charm is deceitful, and beauty is fleeting, but a woman who fears the Lord is to be praised. Give her the reward she has earned and let her works bring her praise at the city gates".

Now wasn't that so nice? Now here's the problem I've always had with this. We were always taught about her, but not how to become a woman like her. Meaning, examples for the modern-day woman. Also, I found that many Christian woman thought just because they were Christian, it automatically made them a virtuous woman. This is far from the truth. Virtuous woman are not born, they are made.

Just like every girl grows up to be a woman, not every woman is a lady. The Proverbs 31 woman was described as a successful entrepreneur of several businesses and a praised wife. She was the perfect woman to study. After receiving my award and having an ah-ha moment, I decided to give it my best shot at breaking this thing down. The principles that I'm about to share with you will can serves as a guide to becoming a better you first. Secondly, it will help you position yourself to be an asset to your Mr. Right aka what I call a Purpose Mate. Disclaimer: You may not agree with everything that I share, but as I was always told, "Eat the meat and spit out the bones." I'm sure you will pick up a few nuggets that will help transform in an Asset Woman.

CHAPTER 1

Femininity

I would be remiss if I didn't start with how vital embracing your femininity will be in this process. You won't be able to use the other valuable keys to their fullest potential if you don't understand the importance of feminine energy. First and foremost, I am not here to tell you that femininity must look a particular way or has a thousand rules. For example, you don't have to wear makeup, the color pink, or love flowers to be feminine. You can very much be feminine without those things. Also, it doesn't make you feminine because you cook, clean or put on dresses either. Those things can totally enhance your femininity, but they don't make you feminine. Short and simple, femininity is about being who you authentically are at your core; being free to live, free to love, free to receive love, and free to just be you.

I read a quote by James E. Faust that said,

"Femininity is the divine adornment of humanity. It finds expression in your qualities of your capacity to love, your spirituality, your radiance, your delicacy, sensitivity, creativity, charm, graciousness, gentleness, dignity, and quiet strength". Powerful.

Because we've been fed that we are to be strong and handle it all, we have lost the very essence of what makes us strong. It's our femininity. We have been trained to be strong in a masculine energy way. What is masculine energy? Here are a few words that will give you a better understanding of what the masculine and feminine energy looks like.

Masculine Energy:

Hunter, protector, provider, aggressive, differentiating, individual, external focus, results-oriented, competitive, action, logic, assertive, cause, and effect, bottom line oriented.

Feminine Energy:

Surrendering, nurturing, catering, values, sensuality, radiant, gentle, tender, patience, loving, empathy intuition, heart, listening, open, accommodating, respond, subconscious, flow, affectionate, receptive, detailed, internal focus, whole focus, planning, giving, being, and focus on efficiency.

These are just a few words that describe the difference between the masculine and feminine.

Because many of us have been thrust into a position to be the provider, it has thrown us into the make it happen grind and hustle mode. As well as our competitive nature has been kicked up to the tenth power in the same manner as a man. It's become our survival mechanism. All the go, go, go, has caused wear and tear on our bodies, mental breakdowns, anxiety and health issues, especially in our womb area. We are so stressed out in our day to day lives that we've learned how to function inside of the dysfunction. There comes the point where you must stop, yes, stop everything and put you first. I know that can be challenging with all the responsibilities that you have on your plate, but if you aren't well how can you help others?

When we operate from masculine energy, we spend much of our time doing and not feeling, connecting with others, taking vacations, or even relaxing. When I say relax I'm not talking about a trip to the nail salon for a Mani-Pedi. I'm talking about getting away from the familiar and doing something spontaneous. When we operate with more masculine energy, we act like we can't live without electronic gadgets, tablets, laptops, and smartphones. We rarely use our creativity and spend time bonding with nature.

When the feminine is underutilized, you will always feel as if there something missing. You will feel a longing for something exciting, refreshing, new, spontaneous, and just some freedom. When your femininity has been lying dormant for a long time, something happens that triggers the longing inside of you, but you can't identify the feeling. It's called the feminine awakening. The funny thing is you, might not even know what it is, but because of how women are wired you're subconsciously seeking what's naturally a part of who you are.

Here are a few ways to embrace your femininity:

1) Stop and Reflect – We have become so busy and routine that we don't pay attention to what's going on, especially what's happening on the inside of us. Have you ever taken the time to pay attention to how you live daily? Day in and day out it's the same thing. You can start to change this by paying attention to how you feel, to be intentional about everything, to think about what you're actually thinking about. I know you're like, "What does she mean by that?". Well, I'm sure you know most of our mood changes are based on what we are thinking about and focusing on. Example, have you ever been having a good day then out of nowhere the thought of what someone did to you, the hurt, or how you were mishandled in the past comes to mind? Then suddenly you get upset, your chest gets tight, and you lose your appetite like it happened at that moment. Now you're walking around in a funk because of what you're thinking about. Another example is music. Music can have this type of effect on your mood as well. Here's an example, we all know what setting the mood means. What is one of the essential tools used to set the mood? That's right, romantic music. No matter how bad of a day you've had, if you come home and your husband has set the mood, your entire disposition will change. So, it's essential that you pay attention to what's on your mind at all times. It's challenging at first, but it becomes natural the more you tune in with yourself.

2) Tap Into Your Emotions- The female and her femininity are conveyed through emotions and feelings. The male and his masculinity are expressed through physical strength and logic. Because of how women are wired, we tend to funnel everything through our emotions. Whereas with men, everything is funneled through logic and facts. Both men and women have emotions, but most of us haven't been taught how to understand and use them. The best way to learn and how to get familiar with yourself is to pay close attention to how you feel. As you start identifying how you're feeling, you automatically begin to feel connected to self.

3) Take Some Me Time- Work, home, school, kids (if you have them) and everything else in between. It's time for you to get out of that routine. If you feel stuck and don't know how to break free, maybe you need some spontaneity in your life. The saying goes "live a little," but I say live a lot. Think about it, you only get one life, no do-overs, no second chances, just one life. It's time to stop existing and live. Try something you've never done before. If money is funny head on over to Groupon or Amazon Deals for some discounted activities. Yes, it will feel weird stepping outside of your comfort zone, but you can't grow being comfortable. Schedule some me time for yourself, daily. I understand your like "April, how can I do that when I have so much to do every single day?" Honey it's called prioritizing. How can you be a benefit to others and you're not a benefit to yourself? Girl stop playing and let go of the guilty feelings that you feel when you take care of yourself. If you don't put you first, who will?

4) **Force Yourself to Change**- Some people think of the feminine as being rejuvenating and quiet, but this is just half the story. It's female energy that alerts you when a shift needs to take place and change needs to happen in your life. This feeling is spectacular. While this process of transformation can feel frightening and wild sometimes, it's required. In the end, we are changing all the time. It is easy to lose touch with your feminine side, but it's an essential part of who you are. Therefore, doing your work to get in touch with who you are at your core is so important. Will it take daily practice and action? Yes. Will it be worth it? Absolutely. You must be willing to go through the emotional pain that comes with change.

CHAPTER 2

Organization

As I studied the Proverbs 31 Woman, I said to myself, "Wow she has a full plate. I wonder how she does it all?". In my mind the only sensible answer would be, she was organized. Think about it; she woke up early, cooked for her family and her maidservants. Her husband was taken care of and her day was pretty much spent on her business endeavors. There was no way that she could have done all those things, and efficient at them if she wasn't organized. The good book says that she was eager to get her day started. I believe she was ready because she had an action plan in place.

I remember back in 2007 when my middle son was about 10. He was such a busybody. Up and down the stairs, inside, outside, wanting to play every few minutes, just an active child. I took it upon myself to create a schedule for him. The chart had a list of times and activities. When the spirit of busyness would come upon him, I would say, "William, it's 5:36, tell me what you should be doing at this very moment." He would shout out, "It says that I'm supposed to be reading between 5:30 and 6." So off he went to get back on task. I saw how effective the schedule was for him, I decided to create one for myself and for my business. I would get excited about new projects and ideas, but not good at following through to completion. I guess William got the spirit of distraction from his mom. From 2007 until today, I still live by the same schedule. Now that the children have left the nest, I fill that time with other things.

Here is an example of what my schedule looked like when the kids were smaller.

5:30 to 6 – Wake up, meditate, and read.

6 to 6:30 – Tidy up and take out what I would cook for dinner. I'm a busy woman, but I usually cooked three to four times a week. I saved a lot of money that way.

6:30 to 7:45 - Getting the kids up and off to school.

7:45 to 8:45 – Finishing up my cleaning and paying bills online. Make personal phone calls like doctors and dentist appointment.

8:45 to 9:45 - Off to the gym. I would take my clothes for the day with me, so I didn't have to get dressed at home. I would just get dressed at the gym and head straight over to my office.

10am to 2:45pm – At the Office.

3 to 3:15pm – Pick up my youngest son.

3:20 to 5pm – Back to the office.

5pm – Head home.

5pm to 7 – Family dinner and homework time.

7:30 to 8 – Kids' bath-time.

8 – 8:30 - Kids' free time.

8:30 to 9 – Kids' bedtime.

9pm – is mom time.

I know it sounds like a lot, but it was effective. I'm also programmed to only work Monday - Thursday 10 to 6 and Fridays 9 to 12 or if at all.

One way to get your day-to-day routine organized is by using your smartphone. You can set your alarm to go off at specific times during the day as a reminder. You've paid enough for that phone, put it to some productive use. Another thing you can do to get organized is to declutter. Yes, I said declutter, and that means all the old clothes, magazines, papers and things you know you will never use. I'm a firm believer that how you feel on the inside will come through on the outside. Ask yourself these questions: Is my home junky? Is my closet a mess? Do I have drawers full of junk mail and papers? Is my car junky? Does my trunk look like a tornado hit it? Does my purse look like I carry my entire house in there? I mean like, cookies and cracker crumbs at the bottom, mixed with safety pins, loose gum, quarters and earring backs.

Ladies, I'm just saying. Do you keep old makeup that you know you will never use? Girl, you know that foundation doesn't match, so let it go. My closet used to look like an earthquake, tornado, and a hurricane hit it. My kids would say that I was a borderline hoarder. There are tons of books and free resources, online, to help you declutter your home. A few things you can do to get started is, go through old clothes that you know you'll never wear again. You can either give them away or make some extra cash by selling them.

CHAPTER 3

Service

―――――◇――――――

"No matter how busy one is, any human being can assert his personality by seizing every opportunity for spiritual activity. How? By his second job. By means of personal actions on however small a scale but the good of his fellow man. He will not have to look far for opportunities". ~ Albert Schweitzer

Proverbs 31:20 says, *"She opens her arms to the poor and extends her arms to the needy."* I am a true believer in being the miracle that someone needs. We get so caught up in our problems that we forget about our neighbor. The best piece of advice that I was given is this. When you're going through your own hardships, the best thing you can do is help someone else. Community work and assisting others is a huge part of my life. Not only does it help those receiving, but it also increases your compassion.

Every year I make an effort to go back and serve the women and children at the homeless shelter where I lived in 2000. If I can't make it back to California, I'll give back right here in Atlanta. I know what it's like to not have a home, car, job, or money. I also remember the feeling of standing in the grocery store checkout line with vouchers holding up the line while people behind me were huffing and puffing. It's very embarrassing and can make you feel worthless like an unfit mother.

I am so grateful for those who extended help in my time of need, as well as an encouraging word. Today, I purchase groceries for others who find themselves in the checkout line experiencing the same embarrassment. Every chance I get, I will buy the food for the car behind me in the drive-through. I started this after someone did it for me. One morning I was going through a few emotional challenges, I felt forgotten and alone. After dropping the kids off at school, I stopped by a local fast food drive-through for some breakfast.

When I pulled up to the window, the cashier said, "The car in front of you paid for your food and said to tell you God bless you, He sees you, and be encouraged." That seemingly small gesture was all I needed to keep going. From that point on I adopted the same form of giving back. You never know what a person needs to hear to keep the faith. We all need to know that someone cares and that we are not alone.

As an Asset Woman, your job is to bring value to the lives of others. I challenge you to contact organizations, check out your neighborhoods and schools to see how you can be of service. Also, another option is to gather some friends, family or the kids and go out and help those living on the streets. Make bag lunches, hold a drive and collect clothes, socks, shoes, and coats. When you look outside of yourself, this is where your blessing happens. I'm often asked, why do you give so much of your time and self to others? I enjoy giving the gift of hope.

There is also another part of giving that you may not be aware of. Are you ready for the secret of getting your breakthrough? Here it is, the more you give, the more abundance you attract into your life. The more I gave, the more I received. The more I took the focus off of my problems, my issues started to seem small and worked themselves out. Even if you don't have finances to give, you can always give of your time and talent. It's your heart and intentions that matter. Do what you can, and I promise it will make someone's day. We are to love our neighbors as we love ourselves. So, ask yourself, "If I were in a time of need would I want someone to come and give me encouraging words? Would I want someone to come and let me know that I can overcome too?"

CHAPTER 4

Finances

Proverbs 31:16 it says *"She considers a field and buys it out of her own earnings she plants a vineyard."* This would suggest that she was confident in her finances. She wasn't worried about her credit, if her ATM card would go through, or if she had to move money from one account to the next. With that said, honestly ask yourself where do I stand financially? Do I have money put away for a rainy day? Am I living from paycheck to paycheck? Am I living beyond my means? Could my credit use some improving? If I lost my job today, would I lose my home/apartment, car, or other possessions in a 30 to 60-day period? Let's be honest, when we tend to judge men, we look at their ability to provide. However, are we what we're asking for? Is our credit as good as what we require of them? Like the title of the book says, 'Being a Woman Who Brings More to the Table Than Her Appetite.'

Being responsible with your finances says a lot about who you are. I know divorce, job loss, not being educated on financial literacy, and setbacks happen. They can cause us to get off track. We've all been there, but we aren't supposed to stay there.

No more hiding from creditors, telling the children to lie and say, "mom isn't home," and no more ignoring the big elephant in the room. First things first, get a copy of your credit report. This is an important step in auditing your finances. After that, start measuring where you stand, add up all your assets such as house, car, stocks, checking, savings account, mutual funds, etc... Do the same with your liabilities like personal loans, credit card debt, student loan, car loan, etc... Now subtract your total liability from the asset amount, and this is your net worth. If your net worth is low or negative, you need to increase your income and decrease your spending. The next question would be "How do I increase my income? Do I need to take on a part-time job?". Starting a business helped me increase my net worth and allowed me to afford the lifestyle and retirement that's important to me. In 2018, it doesn't take a lot of money to start a business, so don't get discouraged.

Here are some tips to help you make some extra cash for savings and to pay off debt.

- Have a garage sale.

- Check out stores that purchase gently used clothing and shoes.

- Write a list before you go to the grocery store, this way you can buy what you need.

- Instead of fast food and microwavable dinners, cook healthy dishes that you can use as leftovers. A little preparation on a Sunday can be well worth it and can leave you with some cheap and easy dinner or snack options for the following week.

- Pull out or invest in a crockpot. This will not only save you money but time as well. Plan your meals around your grocery store flyers.

- Look at the what's on sales, then make recipes based on those ingredients. Do that for a few months, and you'll find how much money that you've saved.

- Cancel unused memberships and subscription services.

- Try generic brands

- Style your own hair

- Do your own Mani and Pedis.

These sacrifices won't be forever, but until you get back on track. Use the 10-second rule. When you pick up a product stop for 10 seconds, look at it, and ask yourself "Is this a need or a want?" If it's a need, get it. If it's a want, put it back. The time will come when you will be able to splurge a little more, but right now it is not that time. You have a goal in mind.

Check out free local events for entertainment. If you must spend a little cash on entertainment, check out Groupon's for great discounts. This next suggestion may not be popular, and it may make you cringe just a little bit, but it's something you may want to consider. Have you ever thought about downsizing? Yes, downsizing. I know it's a sacrifice, but it wouldn't be forever. Look at how much you're spending in rent, taxes, and other expenses. Can you really afford to live where you're currently living? Or would it be more economical to move to a closer city nearby, another state; or, hey, maybe even another country. Who knows, the goal is to get you back on track by any means necessary. Some of the benefits of downsizing are less stress, more money to pay off debt, more leisure and a better mental state, because you're not always full of anxiety and stressed out. So, like I said, I know downsizing may not be the first thing on your mind, but darling always remember change is good. You never know what may happen when you open your mind and heart up to something different.

CHAPTER 5

Class

An asset woman is also a classy woman, the two go hand in hand. I believe the Proverbs 31 woman was a class act as well. After taking a more in-depth look into her life, I see class and elegance written all over it. Conventionally, classy means to be fashionable, refined, tasteful, respectable, gentle and graceful. Nevertheless, I discovered the conventional definition although great descriptions, are a tad limiting. Let's look at some other qualities.

A classy woman is authentic, sincere, of high quality, good character, she holds herself with high standards regardless of what others think of her. She's a woman who doesn't look down on others and gossip. She handles criticism with grace and not in the business of what is now called 'reading' someone. A classy woman will never allow herself to be taken out of character. She sets the atmosphere when she walks into a room, and you can feel the energy shift when she departs. She has an inward glow that goes beyond beauty. A classy woman is not perfect, but she knows how to forgive herself and will aim for better the next time. A classy woman is confident in all that she does. She can handle herself in all social settings, and she is full of smiles.

Today, smiling has become a lost art. Have you ever been told by a man, "smile sweetheart, It can't be that bad?" It's because you're walking around with a sour face. Yup, that face that looks like you just tasted a lemon. It's important to be aware of how you present yourself to the world. Just because you're having some challenges or a bad day, you shouldn't wear how you feel on your face.

One of the hardest things for a woman to accept is a compliment. As I stated before, we are great at giving to others, but we cringe when it's time to receive. Learn how to just say thank you.

Years ago I complimented my mother on her shoes, and the first thing she said was, "I got these from payless for $9.99." I didn't ask her how much she paid for them, I just gave her compliment. Why are women uncomfortable accepting compliments? You cringe at the sound of "that's a pretty dress, you're beautiful, you have pretty eyes." Learn how to sit back, smile and politely say "thank you." A classy woman doesn't downplay herself, she kindly accepts the compliment.

Ok, can I be honest? One of my non-classy traits was my ability to do a lot of yelling. My children would say I would yell all the time and about everything. Yelling is not lady-like. Now that I think about it, why was I yelling anyway? At that time in my life I was miserable and frustrated. The slightest discomfort in my life would set me off. We can't take our frustration out on people that have nothing to do with how we feel. This isn't fair to them, and your words can honestly scar others for a long time. If you find yourself yelling a lot ask yourself,

What am I screaming about?

Will yelling change it?

Why am I frustrated?

Why do I feel the need to yell to get my point across?

Can I ask you something else? Are you gossiper or deal with jealousy? Gossiping and talking negatively about others only shows how you feel about yourself. Love the skin you're in. Yes, there will always be women who are more attractive, smarter and have better bodies than you in your opinion. Does that make you less than? Absolutely not. Why? Because you're an asset, one of a kind and have so much to offer. Loving everything about yourself is the key to walking in confidence, class, and attracting people into your life who will love you on the level that you love yourself. Comparing yourself to others is your biggest enemy. You are made uniquely intentionally, so embrace that.

Love yourself! Love yourself! Love yourself! I always tell my coaching clients that the way you value yourself will determine how you do everything in life.

Everything! If you have a poor view and low value for yourself, so will others. If you don't think you're good enough, others won't either. If you believe that you can't, or you're not lovable or likable, you won't be. I know a lot of this stems from things that happened in your life; traumas, words that were spoken over your life, being mishandled, but it's okay. You forgive, live and move forward. Those things are in the past. Don't let the words, opinions, and actions of others paralyze you. We will always recreate our history by what we're currently focusing on. If you continue to think about what happened in the past, the past will seem to follow you. If you choose to let it go, there is a beautiful future waiting for you on the other side.

Another thing to consider is this. A classy woman wears age appropriate clothing. In the world of twerking and bathroom booty selfies, please have enough respect for yourself to dress in a way that you want to be addressed. You can't get upset with a man for approaching you disrespectfully; if you're disrespecting yourself. I know it's a double standard, but guess what, there will always be a double standard. It is what it is.

CHAPTER 6

Independence

————◆○◆————

Okay, clutch your pearls girls. Women seem to get very upset when I state that we should not live by the "I'm a strong independent woman" mantra. I believe that just because we can or have been put in a position to do it alone, it doesn't mean it was designed to be that way. You see, when you continue to state how independent you are, the energy that comes with that is that you don't need anything or anyone. Yet at the same time and out of the same mouth, you'll say I want and need a man. How can you want a man and want to be independent at the same time? I don't think people really understand the power that words, and thoughts have. Saying you're independent brings you exactly that, being alone and by yourself. This doesn't just work when it comes to relationships, but it works in all areas. Have you ever felt like no one is ever there to come to your aid when you needed them? Yet, everyone can always seem to depend on you when it's their time of need? That's because you're screaming, "I'm independent. I don't need anything. I don't need anyone." So, you're getting exactly that girl. I believe a woman should be able to take care of herself. I just suggest we use the word self-sufficient instead of independent.

Being independent also takes you out of the feminine role. A feminine woman sits back and welcomes help. She views herself as delicate, so she isn't trying to put extra wear, tear, and stress on herself or body. She knows that asking for help and receiving it does not make her look weak. When you live as an independent woman, you should not say what a man should and should not do for you. Why? Because you don't need him anyway. You're independent, right? It's time to start getting what you want by changing your words and actions.

Trust me, you can relinquish control. Oosps, did I say that? I bet you didn't know you were a control freak, huh? I take steps daily to not be one. I now give people the opportunity to help me. In the beginning, it was a little hard, but now it gets easier day-by-day when I accepted that I don't have to do it all. You don't have to prove anything to anyone. I put myself in a position for men to be able to come to my aide. Between you and I, I honestly like being a damsel in distress.

Think about this, have you ever noticed a man will always come to the aid of the woman that has nothing on you, but acts helpless?

Then you wonder why they don't come to your rescue in the same way. It's because you act like Ms. I Got It. One day I was in desperate need of $750 for my rent. A male friend called and asked how I was doing. I told him I needed the money by 3 PM, and could he help. He gave me some encouraging word and said I was smart and I would figure it out.

Another young lady that he viewed as a damsel in distress had the same need that I had. Guess what he did? Yep, he figured out a solution for her. That made me feel some kind of way. I asked him, what was it about her that made him fix her problem? He said that I was a strong woman and could figure anything out. From that point on, I learned how to be vulnerable, and show a man that I didn't have it all together. If you think about it, it's not game playing because I really didn't have it together. Vulnerability helped me get back in the feminine position of receiving.

When you look at the Proverbs 31 woman, she had maidservants. This would suggest that she recognized that she needed help. Long gone are the days of trying to do it all alone. I'm not straining my back, my knees, or my brain trying to prove that I can be superwoman. I've officially taken my cape off. We end up with all kinds of aches and pains because we're trying to do everything for everyone and still end up feeling empty and unhappy.

CHAPTER 7

Health

I'm going to address something that is not necessarily talked about in the story, but it stuck out to me. Based upon all the responsibilities the Proverbs 31 woman had, I believe it's safe to say she was healthy and fit.

You don't have to be a size two, but you should want to be healthy for your body type. I believe she would not have been able to accomplish her daily task if she didn't practice good health. Think about it, it says that she gets up early in the morning, cooks for her family and enough for her maidservants, she helps the poor, runs several businesses, takes care of her husband,

and the list goes on. It even says her arms were strong, and she sets about her work vigorously. Honey, I'm tired just thinking about it. There is no way you can do all of that, and not have some type of fitness regimen. No, we don't always want to work-out because of the time and effort it requires. The last thing we need is to have to get up and get on a treadmill when we have so much to do, and so little time. It's even been said that the main reason African-American women don't like to work out is because we don't want to mess up our hair. It's a little shallow, but I've heard it quite a bit. I don't know about you, but I would rather mess up my hair than have a heart attack.

Heart disease is the number one killer of women. I'm going to assume that in addition to having some type of fitness regimen, she probably cooked healthy meals. Listen, I love cake, pies, ice-cream, and a brownie just like everyone else. I'm what you call a dessert connoisseur, pound cake is my favorite. However, I can't complain about feeling sluggish, down, tired, fatigued, having a lack of energy because I am pumping all if this crap into my body. To be more productive, you need to put the right foods in your body. I know fast food seems like a quick and convenient option, but is it really?

Not long ago I found myself sick. Didn't know what was going on, I found that I was having digestive issues. I was then told I had fibroids. I started doing some research on my own and decided to change my diet. It was a challenge because I didn't know exactly where to start, so I called a friend who is a vegan chef. She came over with a folder filled with paper. My thought was, "Oh my God what is all of this? Since when did eating right require stacks of papers?" Long story short, she took me to the grocery store, and we were there for two hours. We walked row by row, aisle by aisle and she said, "April, everything you see on the shelves called food products. It's not actually real food." She went on to say, "If you can't pronounce what's on the back, put it back." I stood there shocked and said, "wait, wait, wait, hold on. So, you mean to tell me that my mac and cheese out of the box, my crackers, and all of my other goodies, are food products?" She said, "Yes, they are not living food. You have manufacturers who make a lot of money creating food products".

At that moment, I knew I had to make some changes. Still, in shock about this new-found knowledge, I said, "so, you mean to tell me my Peanut Butter Captain Crunch and Cinnamon Toast Crunch are all manufactured food products?". She simply said "yes." Row by row, aisle by aisle, we went on this field trip picking up my favorites and saying to myself, "April you cannot pronounce what's on the back of any of this stuff." Out of frustration, I asked her, "Well what do we eat?"

I mean I almost had a breakdown in the freezer section. We like the frozen pizzas and the quick frozen dinners, but the more we explored the aisles, the more I realized the amount of junk I had been putting in my body.

As I stood there having a tantrum I asked once again "What in the world are we supposed to eat, because I'm standing here and I'm about to cry, and I have no idea what I'm going to do, so what do you mean I have to clean out my cabinets. What am I going feed my kids? You know I'm just having a breakdown, right?" She says, "If you are a living being you should be eating living foods." Then she says, "If you were stuck on a desert island would you pick up the dead chicken that you see and eat it, or would you pick up the live apple?" That was a no-brainer, I'd pick up the live apple. She said, "Exactly! So why would you go to the grocery store and buy a dead chicken to eat?" At that moment I I understood, and a light bulb came on. I tried going vegan for a little while. It wasn't totally for me, but I did notice some changes. I'm not saying you should cut everything out all at one time, but I am saying moderation is vital.

After that experience, I really understood the importance of health. I never paid attention to it so much because we are always on the go and take our bodies for granted. We think that we'll always have the privilege of getting out of bed, taking care of myself, but that is not necessarily true. So, ask yourself, have I been neglecting my health? What kind of food do I eat daily? As they say, breakfast is the most important meal. Do you eat a healthy breakfast every day? Do you eat 5-6 times a day? Do you look in the mirror and say, I hate the way that I look, but do nothing about it? Instead of working out you know what we do, we buy contraptions like waist trainers, girdles, butt lifters, waist centers, push this up, push that down, smash that in, etc.... The beauty is a billion dollar industry.

One reason for this is, instead of wanting to do the work, we would rather buy products that will conceal and make them look smaller, feel sexier, instead of doing the work to become smaller or sexier. Trust me I know! I have a waist trainer too. But it wasn't until I took responsibility that I stated to make changes. I wanted to put on a cute little summer or spring dress without feeling like I'm in a straitjacket.

You might be thinking that you don't have time. Do we ever have time, or do we make time? I've always been told we make time for what we deem is important to us. Our health needs to be more of a priority. Here are some things that I did to get myself back on track. I am an early riser, and I have a set of videos in my playlist on YouTube that I follow several times a week. Although you may not have a gym membership, you can't let that stop you and be an excuse. I also, get up and walk around the tennis court. There are so many free resources online, you'll just have to make the decision to use them.

CHAPTER 8

Faith

As I continued my own journey of self-discovery, I understood just how vital my spirituality and faith would be.

I began to love faith when I learned how to use it. What is faith? It's the substance of things hoped for, the evidence of things not seen. Another way to put it is; having complete trust, confidence, and loyalty in something without having to see it. You see, there are so many times we desire something in our lives, but we don't have enough faith to believe that we can have it. It sounds good to say, "Yes, I can have it all", but do we really believe that we can have better health, wealth, peace, love and abundance? We say we believe, but sometimes I really don't think that we do. When you have faith in something what you are saying is, no matter what I see, I will not waiver. No matter how dark times get, I will not be moved. No matter how fear, depression, and anxiety try to take over me, I refuse to stop believing that I can create the life I desire

Worry stops when you believe. When you have faith, you do what you can and let God or the universe do the rest. When you have faith, there is a calm and peacefulness of knowing that things are already okay. Not they will be okay, but they are ok. Think about this, when you know that you're good at something you just know it, and there's nothing anyone else can tell you. This is because you have faith in your abilities. Now, of course, the enemy of faith is fear. Yes, fear will come, but there is something you must remember. Fear is something that only you can create in your mind. Isn't that interesting? You can choose to have faith, or you can choose to have fear.

I'm here to tell you that you can choose what you think, what you believe, and how you feel? Whatever you decide is what it will be.

When I started to understand this better, that is when I fell in love with executing my faith and manifestation.

Fear is nothing more than ideas, scenarios, and situations that you create in your mind. Most of the things that you're afraid of have never happened. We put ourselves in a state of panic. We play a part in creating our own anxiety by continually replaying the negatives. We play out scenarios that always end up with an adverse outcome. We still play the "what if" game, but we play it negatively. It's time for you to change what you know and how you think. Just like you can play the "what if" in an adverse scenario, you can play it with a positive outcome. Think of it like this. What if it does work? What if I can be healthy? What if I can meet the love of my life? What if I can start a successful business? Catch my drift? Just like you can

.

have faith in the negative you can have faith in the positive. The choice is yours darling.

Also, please, please, please remember, whatever you think of the most and add feeling to is what will manifest in your life. Let me say that again. Whatever you think on the most and add feeling to is what you will manifest in your life. Do you remember when you were younger, and someone did something hurtful to you? It really pierced you to your core. Now let's fast forward years later when you hear those same words or think about what happened. You can still fill the sting and emotions will rise as though it happened in that moment. Words have life and they're still living on the inside of you. What you've done is placed feeling onto those words, which means you continue to recreate those same scenarios in your life.

I remember I would wake feeling like I would get pulled over by the police that day. I just knew the police were going to stop me and give me a ticket. I would play how the entire interaction would go in my mind. How negative, right? Well, sure enough, I would get pulled over. Yep, I created that reality with my thoughts.

At that time, I didn't know that I could change those feelings and thoughts. I could've easily turned those thoughts and feeling into something positive like, "today is a great day, and everything is going to go my way. I live in abundance and grace."

Here is another example of how I used my faith (without realizing it) to manifest my desires.

One day I wanted a slice of pound cake. I craved some pound cake to the point I could see it, smell it, and I could even taste it. I wanted it like the air that I needed to breathe. The very next day I went to the hair salon, and you'll never guess what happened. A woman walked in with a basket and said, "would anyone like to buy some pound cake?". Can you imagine how shocked I was? I literally created what I wanted, and it came to me. That pound cake seemed like the best piece of cake I'd ever had.

I was able to manifest a slice of cake because I could smell it, taste it and see it like it was right in front of me. I had no doubt, nor did I try to rationalize why I should not have it. I set my intention and left it alone. Like I said, you can create abundance in your life, or you can create lack in your life. The determining factor has everything to do with how you think, what believe and how you feel about those things. I have a more in-depth course with the exact steps you need to alter your life. The title is 'Manifest - *How to Change the Way You Think To Manifest The Life, Love & Abundance You Desire.*' You can visit www.aprilmason.com to download the course.

CHAPTER 9

Wisdom

A s women, we are extremely emotional. Many times, to our detriment we don't think before we speak. However, there comes a time when you must use wisdom. Wisdom is something that allows you to know when to talk and when to be silent. Now don't get me wrong, being sweet does not equal weak or makes you a doormat. We will often put our foot in our mouth because our emotions are out of control, and we just want to speak how we feel at that moment. I've seen on shows like Divorce Court or Judge Judy where she might have been in favor of the woman, but because she could not be quiet and had the 'I just have to tell it' attitude she loses everything. There are times in life that you must learn how to hush, as my Grandfather would say. You can allow your emotions to talk you right out of a good thing. Be it in business, romantic relationships, on the job and friendships.

I've read a lot of books on business, and one thing majority of them had in common is, knowing when to listen. If you listen, people will tell you everything that you need to know.

When my son had issues in school with his mouth, I would tell him, "son you never want to win the battle and lose the war."

You see we get a high out of being able to release our emotions in a matter that makes us feel empowered. That usually consists of getting loud, angry, talking fast, and spewing out whatever comes to mind. But here is the big question, what did you gain? Nothing more than a feeling of release. Something like a woo-sah because you were able to get it off your chest and mind, but you still didn't get the resolution that you were after. If your head is in the lion's mouth, you rub the lions head until you get it out. This applies to relationships as well as your day-to-day life, especially at your place of employment. Companies would have less in-house drama if more people used wisdom.

Ladies, it would behoove you to learn how to use wisdom in everything you do. You don't always have to prove your point or give your opinion. Especially on things that will not affect you either way. I'm not suggesting that you don't speak up for yourself.

I'm merely saying that how you do it, and asking yourself, " does this situation warrant a response?" should be your first thought before you respond.

When my children were smaller, they would do typical kid stuff that would get them in trouble. What would I do? Get quiet. I'll never forget my daughter being in her bedroom with her brothers, and I overheard her tell them,

"You guys don't get it yet, do ya?" And Cory says, "What do you mean Adri?" "Have you noticed that when Mom says, Really? Okay, mmm hmm, and gets quiet, that means we're really in trouble?".

They would go into overdrive trying to make things right because they knew there was something lethal in my silence. When you are silent, people can't gauge which direction you're going to go in.

You should also use wisdom when it comes to the people you choose to put in your life and how you handle situations that arise. Kick up that discerning spirit - that woman's intuition. Use wisdom in the decisions that you make every single day. Wisdom and knowing how to apply it is your best friend.

Being smart is knowing that a tomato is a fruit. Wisdom is knowing not to add it to a fruit salad. -Author Unknow

CHAPTER 10

Entrepreneurship

Cha-ching!

In this chapter, I'm going to discuss the importance of finances. As the story is told, the Proverbs 31 woman was a successful entrepreneur. I've a been a full-time entrepreneur for 15 years now. There have been many ups and downs, but I wouldn't change it. The freedom I have is priceless, and it allows me to do what I love and live a balanced life. Not to mention, I was able to pay off debt and invest. Every woman does not have the entrepreneurial bug, and that doesn't make you less of an Asset Woman.

However, although you may be content working in Corporate America, I urge you to always have other sources of income coming in. This doesn't mean you have to operate a full-time business, it just means to think about the future. I believe that every woman should have at least six months' worth of emergency funds available. Life happens, and the worse feeling is when life does happen, and money if funny too.

As an Asset Woman, it's imperative that you bring in more income to pay off debtors and add to your savings. It can be challenging to decrease debt and save when you're only making enough to take care of your day to day necessities. If you aren't ready or not sure if you want to take the entrepreneurial leap, here are a few ways to bring in some extra cash.

1) Sell items that you know longer use on eBay, craigslist, or have a garage sale. There are also several apps that you can download on your phone to sell your goods.

2) Rent your home or apartment on Airbnb.

3) If you have a car or a second car that you don't use much, rent it out on Turo.

4) Invest in stocks

5) Drive for Uber or Lyft in your spare time

These are only a few ideas of what you can do to earn some extra money. If you do an online search for "how to make extra money," tons of other ideas will pop up. At this point, you have to decide to get intentional about your financial future.

Now if you are ready to start a business, but don't know where to start, let's start at the beginning. In my opinion, one of the best ways to decide what type of business to start is by finding your purpose first. Why is this so important? Think of it this way. Have you ever had a friend or family member who was always jumping from business opportunity to business opportunity? One day they are selling tea, legal services, cupcakes and waist trainers. Then in the next two weeks, they ask you to buy vitamins, diet juices, jewelry and the list goes on.

When you haven't found your purpose, you chase anything that you believe will make money. This type of thinking will hurt you in the long run because you won't be invested in it. The goal is to find your purpose in life and learn how to create multiple streams of income from it.

So, your question at this point is, how do I find my purpose April?

Let's start with making sure that you understand that you were born with a unique assortment of gifts, talents, and abilities. You cannot be duplicated because you are one of a kind. Yes, you may see others who can do similar things as you, but no one can do it the way you can.

When you're operating in your life's purpose, your goals and ambitions will have a lot more meaning to you. On the days you want to give up (which will happen), understanding your life's purpose will ignite you and give you the motivation to keep going. At the end of this chapter, I have a list of questions that will help you identify your purpose.

Once you've found your purpose, the next step is to figure out how to create multiple streams of income from it. One way is to create a product or service from what you naturally know. Yes, people will pay you for what you know or can do. You may not value your natural gifts and abilities, but others will. This is where believing in yourself and knowing that you're enough comes in to play. Before I go any further, let me explain what I mean. Often as women, we don't feel like we're enough, worthy, or deserving. This type of belief system not only affects your life, but also how you value your business.

When I had no value for myself, I would complain about not making enough money. It wasn't that I had a bad product or service, it was that my value of myself spilled over into my business. I wasn't charging enough for the results that my services rendered to the client. I would complain about not having money for the light bill, not realize that I was my own hindrance. So, as you see, how you feel about you will cause you not to value what you do. Which in turn will have you afraid of putting a value on what you offer. That's why the previous chapters of this book are so relevant. Becoming an Asset Woman and valuing who you are plays out in the results that you receive across the board. Your view of yourself holds the key to attracting better men, better clients, better career opportunities and even better friendships. It all starts with you. If you want better results, you must become a better woman. The questions below will help you get on the road to discovering your purpose.

1) What do you do well?

2) What do you love to do?

3) What do you do that comes naturally to you?

4) What drives you up the wall?

5) What do people compliment you on?

6) What are your strengths?

7) What makes you feel great about yourself?

8) If you had to teach something, what would it be?

9) What causes do you firmly believe in?

10) What are some challenges, difficulties, and hardships you've overcome or are in the process of overcoming? How did you do it?

11) When you're 90 years old, what do you want to be remembered for?

CHAPTER 11

Self Love

Have you ever noticed that people who mishandle others will not allow anyone to do it to them? They have a double standard of I can do it to you, but I refuse to let you do it to me. This is because of their personal standard and boundaries that they've set for themselves.

It boils down to this, you can choose to love yourself, or you can choose not to. Whichever you select will be right for you.

Here are a few actionable steps that you can take to love yourself more. Carve out thirty minutes of me time per day. I know I discussed this earlier in a previous chapter, but I wanted to reiterate just how important this is. I know it can seems impossible but think about this. When you're watching a television show, it normally lasts 30 minutes to an hour, aren't you worth 30 – 60 minutes? During that time relax, let your worries go, inhale, exhale and just be. Don't try and fix anything, don't think of any projects that you have coming up, the kids, family, friends, none of that. Just enjoy some peace. Reward yourself, show yourself some appreciation, and do something nice for you. Have dinner at a five star restaurant, purchase something that you wouldn't normally buy for yourself.

Now let me talk about that for a moment. One of the exercises that I had one of my private coaching clients do is buy something that's more expensive than she usually spends on herself. She had the hardest time with this exercise.

When I say expensive I'm not talking about thousands. More like, if you usually pay $39 for a pair of shoes, go up to $100 or $150. My client was terffied to do this. One day I received a text message from her, and it was a receipt. She invested $300 in herself. If you have children you know how difficult it can be to treat yourself. Your mind starts to think about all the things the kids may need.

After she texted me what she purchased, I texted her back and said, "Tear up the receipt and send me a screenshot." It took her a minute to do because it was challenging, but she did it. That's something you can try as well.

A few more ideas are to take yourself on a date and take on a new hobby.

This next exercise is to help you reinforce just how awesome you are.

Stand in front of the mirror, pick out the affirmations below that resonates with you, and post them in your bathroom, cubicle at your work, your car and wherever you frequent often. Are you ready to say these affirmations with me? Alright, let's go!

I am lovable.

I am likable.

I am powerful.

I am healthy.

I am smart.

I am funny.

I am successful.

I am a fantastic woman.

I am happy and full of joy.

I am beautiful on the inside and out.

Only I can create the life that I desire.

I put myself first and make no apologies for it.

I take care of myself and well-being.

I love and accept love unconditionally.

I approve of myself.

I feel great about myself.

I love everything about myself including my flaws.

I radiate love and respect, and in return, I receive love and respect.

I am a cultured and wise, yet humble.

My high self-esteem enables me to respect myself.

I make sound and intentional decisions.

I am a unique and extraordinary person, and worthy of love and respect from others.

I will never allow another man to devalue or mishandle me no matter how much I may love or care about him.

My high self-esteem enables me to accept compliments easily and freely give them.

I understand that there is no excuse for anyone to ever treat me poorly.

I accept others as they are and they, in turn they accept me as I am.

I deserve all that is good.

I release any need for misery and suffering.

I release the need to prove myself to anyone.

I am solution minded. Any problem that comes is solvable.

I am never alone, I am always supported.

My mind is filled with only loving, healthy, positive and prosperous thoughts, which ultimately are manifested in my life.

My mind and heart are full of gratitude for my lovely and beautiful life.

My circumstances no longer hold me hostage.

I consciously release the past and live only in the present.

This way I can enjoy and experience life to the fullest.

I am making positive changes in my life.

I choose to make better choices when it comes to my food.

As I change my thoughts, everything around me changes. I am excited about the person I am becoming, and I love me some me.

CONCLUSION

In this quick read, my goal was to provide you with practical tools to give you the courage to redesign your life. You are now equipped to rise up and be the feminine Asset Woman that is long to make her entrance.

If you only take away one thing, take away this. You are meant to live an abundant life. You have the power to create whatever you desire. If you're not sure how, connect with those who are living it. Be it investing in a coach, program, or free resources. When it comes to this life, there are no do-overs. When you apply the keys in this book, you will see the difference in the type of men you attract, how you think, the love you have for yourself, and the possibilities. **You are An Asset!**

OTHER HELPFUL RESOURCES

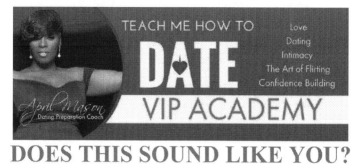

DOES THIS SOUND LIKE YOU?

Has dating become a chore?

Are you successful, educated and beautiful, but can't seem to attract a quality date?

Haven't had a fun, exciting and meaningful date in years?

Do you feel like all the quality men are taken?

Are you wondering if there is even a man out there for you?

Does your masculinity shine through on a date instead of your femininity?

Not sure how to get back out there as an Asset Woman?

VIP ACADEMY MEMBERSHIP INCLUDES
Monthly LIVE Masterclass | Video Dating Tips | Printable Workbook | Printable Weekly Dating Plan | The Asset HOT Seat | Q&A

JOIN TODAY! www.vip.teachmehowtodate.com

NEED PERSONAL ADVICE?

Download the Magnifi app and
call me directly today!

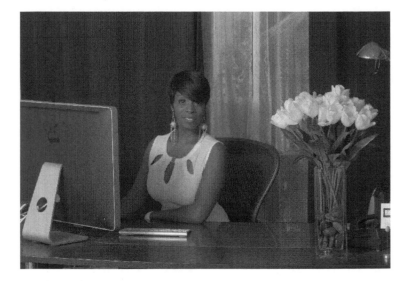

DOWNLOAD TODAY WWW.APRILMASON.COM

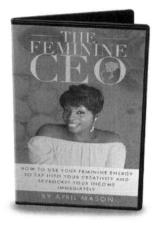

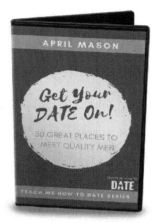

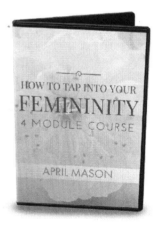

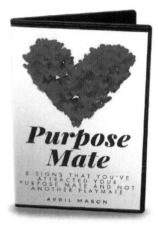

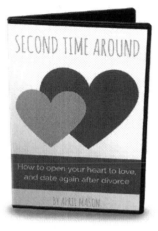

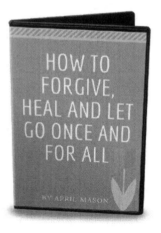

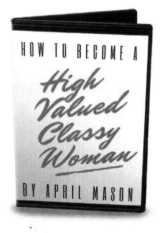

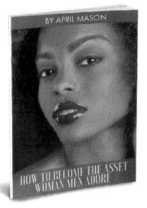

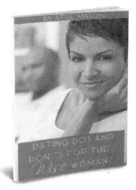

Made in the USA
Middletown, DE
27 December 2019